Copyright 2023

All right reserved. No part of this book should be reproduced without express permission of the author.

Reproduction of all or any part of this book is punishable under relevant law.

Table of Contents

Lymphoma is cancer that begins in infection-fighting cells of the immune system, called lymphocytes. These cells are in the lymph nodes, spleen, thymus, bone marrow, and other parts of the body. When you have lymphoma, lymphocytes change and grow out of control.

There are two main types of lymphoma:

Non-Hodgkin: Most people with lymphoma have this type.

Hodgkin

Non-Hodgkin and Hodgkin lymphoma involve different types of lymphocyte cells. Every type of lymphoma grows at a different rate and responds differently to treatment.

Lymphoma is very treatable, and the outlook can vary depending on the type of lymphoma and its stage. Your doctor can help you find the right treatment for your type and stage of the illness.

Lymphoma is different from leukemia. Each of these cancers starts in a different type of cell.

Lymphoma starts in infection-fighting lymphocytes.

Leukemia starts in blood-forming cells inside bone marrow.

Lymphoma is also not the same as lymphedema, which is a collection of fluid that forms in body tissues when there is damage or blockage to the lymph system.

BREAKFAST

1. Full English Breakfast

Prep Time: 20 Minutes

Cook Time: 45 Minutes

Servings: 2

Ingredients

- 1 large potato, cut into small cubes
- 3 tablespoons olive oil, divided
- 2 teaspoons kosher salt, divided
- 2 teaspoons black pepper, divided
- 1 teaspoon garlic powder
- 1 teaspoon paprika
- 8 strips bacon
- 12 ounces mushrooms, sliced
- 1/ 2 teaspoon red pepper flakes

Fresh lemon juice:

- 2 roma tomatoes, sliced

- 4 slices sourdough bread
- 1 (12 ounce) can baked beans
- 4 eggs
- Fresh chives, finely chopped, for serving

Instructions

1. Preheat oven to 400°F and line a large baking sheet with parchment paper. Pour the potato cubes onto the sheet and drizzle on 1 tablespoon olive oil, 1 teaspoon salt, 1 teaspoon black pepper, 1 teaspoon garlic powder, and 1 teaspoon paprika. Toss to evenly coat, then bake for 45 minutes, or until golden brown and crispy on the outside.

2. Line a second baking sheet with parchment and place the bacon strips onto the parchment, spaced 1 inch apart. Place into the preheated oven to bake for 20-30 minutes, or to your desired doneness.

3. Meanwhile, sauté mushrooms. Heat 1 tablespoon olive oil in a large pan over medium-high heat. Add in mushrooms and cook, stirring frequently, until golden brown. Once nearly done cooking, season with 1/2 teaspoon salt, 1/2 teaspoon black pepper, and 1/2

teaspoon red pepper flakes. Squeeze on some fresh lemon juice, then set mushrooms aside.

4. Next, make the tomatoes. Coat both sides of the tomato slices in olive oil, salt, and pepper. Heat a grill pan or large cast iron skillet over medium-high. Place the tomatoes down onto the pan and cook for about 3 minutes per side. Set aside.

5. In a medium pot over medium heat, gently heat up the baked beans. Toast the pieces of bread to your liking.

6. Heat 1/2 tablespoon olive oil in a large pan over medium-high heat. Crack in 2 eggs and cook until the whites are set, about 5 minutes, for a sunny-side up egg. Repeat for additional 2 eggs if you want more eggs.

7. Plate everything together - roasted potatoes, crispy bacon, sautéed mushrooms, seared tomatoes, baked beans, toast, and fried eggs. Top with fresh chives. Enjoy!

Prep Time: 15 Minutes

Cook Time: 25 Minutes

Servings: 4

Ingredients

For The Pico:

- 3 roma tomatoes, cored and finely chopped
- 1/ 2 cup finely chopped fresh cilantro
- 1/ 4 cup finely chopped red onion
- 1 lime, zested and juiced
- 1 small jalapeño, seeded and diced
- Salt, to taste
- Black peppercorns, freshly ground, to taste

For The Burrito:

- 3 medium Yukon Gold potatoes
- 4 tablespoons La Tourangelle Grapeseed Oil, divided
- 8 ounces spicy chorizo sausage, casings removed
- 1 tablespoon garlic powder
- 1 tablespoon onion powder
- 1/ 2 teaspoon cayenne

- 1 small bunch scallions, ends trimmed and thinly sliced
- 6 large eggs, vigorously whisked
- 4 large tortillas
- 1 avocado, sliced
- 1 cup grated sharp cheddar cheese
- Hot sauce, for serving

Instructions

1. Preheat oven to 350°F.
2. Make the pico: In a medium bowl, combine all ingredients and season to taste. Store in refrigerator.
3. Grate potatoes and transfer to clean kitchen towel, squeezing out any excess liquid. Keep wrapped in kitchen towel.
4. Heat 2 tablespoons grapeseed oil in a cast iron skillet over medium high heat. Cook chorizo, breaking up with a heat proof spatula into small crumbles, until golden brown, about 8 minutes. Remove with a slotted spoon and set aside.
5. In the same skillet, add potatoes. Season with garlic powder, onion powder, cayenne, salt and pepper. Arrange in a single layer across the pan and cook

undisturbed until golden brown, 4 minutes. Flip to brown other sides of potatoes, another 4 minutes. Remove from pan and set aside. Wipe out skillet completely.

6. Reduce heat to medium and heat remaining 2 tablespoons grapeseed oil in skillet. Add scallions and cook until softened, 2 minutes. Add eggs and scramble, about 2 minutes. Remove from skillet and set aside.

7. To assemble burritos, divide egg mixture, chorizo, potatoes, pico, avocado slices, and cheese between 4 tortillas. Tuck sides in and wrap tightly. Arrange burritos on baking sheet. Transfer to oven and cook until cheese is melted, 10 minutes. Halve and serve with hot sauce immediately.

Prep Time: 15 Minutes

Cook Time: 25 Minutes

Servings: 2-3

Ingredients

For The Hash:

- 3 slices thick cut bacon
- 2 tablespoons olive oil or butter, divided
- 1/ 2 large red onion, chopped
- 1 red bell pepper, chopped
- 2 cloves garlic, minced
- 1 1/ 2 cups sweet potato, peeled and diced into 3/4-inch cubes
- 1/ 4 teaspoon salt
- 1 1/ 2 cups kale, de-ribbed and chopped
- 1/ 4 teaspoon black pepper
- 3 large eggs
- Shaved parmesan or feta crumbles, if desired

Instructions

1. Put the three slices of bacon in a large cast iron skillet over medium low heat. Cook until the bacon is browned, about 6 minutes, flipping about halfway through. Once browned and crisped, remove to a plate lined with a paper towel.

2. Add the 1 tablespoon of the oil or butter to the pan with the bacon grease and cook the onion and bell pepper until tender, about 3 minutes. Toss in the garlic and sweet potato and salt, cover the pan, and cook, stirring occasionally, until the sweet potato are tender to a fork, about 15 minutes.

3. In the meantime, chop the bacon and prepare your oats (see below). Once the potato are perfectly cooked, toss in the kale and pepper. Stir just until the kale is wilted and then salt to taste.

4. Remove the vegetables from the pan and add the remaining tablespoon of oil or butter. Crack the eggs into the pan and cover. Cook until the egg whites are opaque and no clear remains, 2-3 minutes. If you prefer your egg yolks a bit more done, continue cooking to your preference. Slip the eggs out of the pan and then assemble your bowls.

5. Divide the oats among 2-3 bowls (depending on your portion preference) and then add the veggies on top. Finish each bowl with an egg and cheese, if desired. Add salt and pepper to taste and enjoy!

For The Oats:

- 2 cups water
- 1 cup quick cooking oats
- 1/ 4 teaspoon salt
- 1 tablespoon prepared basil pesto
- 1/ 8 teaspoon black pepper

Instructions

1. Bring the water to a boil in a small saucepan over medium heat. Add the oats and salt and turn the heat down to medium-low. Cook for about 1 minute, stir in the pesto and pepper, and then set aside of the heat.

Prep Time: 5 Minutes

Cook Time: 30 Minutes

Servings: 12

Ingredients

- 3 cups old fashioned oats
- 1 cup almond flour
- 1 cup canned pumpkin
- 1/ 2 cup maple syrup
- 1/ 2 cup coconut oil
- 1/ 2 teaspoon salt
- 1/ 2 teaspoon baking powder
- 2 teaspoon cinnamon
- 1 teaspoon ground ginger
- 1/ 2 teaspoon cloves
- 1/ 4 teaspoon nutmeg
- 1/ 2 cup dark chocolate chips, optional

Instructions

2. Preheat oven to 350°F. Line baking sheet with parchment paper or spray with cooking spray.

3. Pulse the oats in food processor until roughly chopped. Put in a mixing bowl and mix with all of the other dry ingredients, almond flour, salt, cinnamon, ginger, cloves, and nutmeg.

4. In a separate bowl, whisk all of the wet ingredients together: pumpkin, maple syrup and coconut oil.

5. Fold wet ingredients into dry ingredients and blend. Add chocolate chips if you would like!

6. Use a 1/4 measuring cup to drop the batter onto the baking sheet. Space one inch apart and press down lightly.

7. Bake in the center of the oven for 30-35 minutes or until sides and bottom are golden brown. Allow to cool completely on the sheet pan and then enjoy!

Prep Time: 5 Minutes

Cook Time: 15 Minutes

Servings: 4

Ingredients

- 8 Mini-Waffles, made fresh or heated frozen

Buffalo Sauce

- 1/ 2 cup watercress
- Pickled Green Tomato
- Maple Syrup-Glazed Buttermilk Fried Chicken
- 4 slices Land O Lakes, cut in half

Quick Pickled Green Tomatoes:

- 1 green tomato, sliced about 1/4" thick
- 1 cup apple cider vinegar
- 1 cup water
- 1 garlic clove, minced
- 1 tablespoon salt
- 1 teaspoon black pepper
- 1 tablespoon sugar

Buffalo Sauce:

- 2 tablespoon hot sauce
- 2 tablespoon unsalted butter, melted

Buttermilk Fried Chicken:

- 1 pound chicken tenderloins
- 1/2 cup + 3 tbsp buttermilk
- 1 1/ 2 teaspoon salt
- 1/ 8 teaspoon cayenne pepper
- 1/ 2 teaspoon garlic powder
- 1/ 2 teaspoon paprika
- 3/ 4 cup flour
- 3/ 4 teaspoon baking powder
- 3 cups vegetable oil, for cooking
- 2 tablespoon maple syrup
- 2 tablespoon honey

Instructions

1. In a small bowl, combine the vinegar, water, garlic, salt, pepper, and sugar. Place tomatoes in a shallow bowl or mason jar and pour vinegar mixture on top. Let sit at room temperature for 45 minutes to 1 hour.

For The Buffalo Sauce:

1. Whisk together hot sauce and butter until combined. Set aside.

For The Buttermilk Fried Chicken:

1. Make marinade by combining 1/2 cup buttermilk, 1 teaspoon salt, cayenne pepper, 1/4 teaspoon garlic powder, and 1/4 teaspoon paprika. Combine with chicken tenders in a large resealable bag. Make sure chicken tenders are evenly coated with marinade and refrigerate overnight, or at least 4 hours.
2. Make breading by mixing flour, remaining salt, remaining garlic powder, remaining paprika, flour, and baking powder in a bowl. Once combined, add buttermilk and stir until evenly clumpy.
3. Remove chicken from marinade and coat with flour mixture until the breading sticks to the meat.
4. Heat oil over high heat in a pot (there should be about 1 inch of oil in pot). Once oil is heated, place chicken tenders in oil and cook each side until golden brown, about 1 minute per side. Once cooked, set aside on plates lined with paper towels. Repeat process until all chicken tenders are fried. Cool chicken for a few minutes.

5. While chicken is cooling, whisk together maple syrup and honey in a small bowl. Brush both sides of the chicken with maple syrup mixture.

Assembly:

1. Preheat oven to 400 degrees. Line baking sheet with parchment paper. On baking sheet, brush 8 waffle slices with buffalo sauce, sauce side up. Divide watercress among 4 waffles, about 2 tablespoons per waffle. Place one slice of green tomato on top of watercress. Place 1 piece of chicken on top of tomato. Divide Land O Lakes among the 4 sandwiches and layer on top of chicken. Top with waffle, sauce side down, and stick with food pick. Bake sandwiches in oven for about 3 minutes, or until Deli American melts. Serve immediately.

Prep Time: 10 Minutes

Cook Time: 15 Minutes

Servings: 4

Ingredients

- 3 tablespoon olive oil, divided
- 1 large bunch asparagus, trimmed to 1 inch pieces
- Salt and pepper, to taste
- 4 eggs
- 3 teaspoons lemon juice
- 1/ 2 teaspoon shallot, finely diced
- 1/ 2 teaspoon Dijon mustard
- Salt and pepper, to taste
- 1 avocado
- 1 cup microgreens
- 2 cups arugula
- 1/ 4 cup sunflower seeds

2. Heat the 1 tbsp olive oil in a small pan on medium-high heat. Add the asparagus pieces, season with salt and pepper and cook for 2-4 minutes (depending on the thickness of your stalks). Set aside.

3. Heat a small pot of water on high heat and bring to a boil. Reduce the heat to a gentle simmer and with a spoon, carefully add the eggs. Immediately set a timer for 6½ minutes for soft-boiled eggs. If you'd like your eggs a little firmer, set your timer for 7 - 7½ minutes. Increase the heat until you reach a boil again. While the eggs are boiling, create an ice-water bath in a bowl. When the eggs are done, remove them from the pot with your spoon and immediately submerge in the ice-water bath, to stop the cooking process.

4. Make the lemon vinaigrette by whisking together remaining, 2 tbsp olive oil, lemon juice, shallot, Dijon mustard, salt, and pepper in a small bowl, and set aside.

5. Assemble the salads by dividing up the arugula and microgreens between two bowls. Add the asparagus and sunflower seeds. Peel and slice the avocado, adding a ¼ avocado to each serving. Peel the eggs,

slice in half and add to the salads. Drizzle the lemon vinaigrette on top.

Prep Time: 10 Minutes

Cook Time: 15 Minutes

Servings: 4

Ingredients

- 1 (14.5 ounce) can Muir Glen Organic Whole Peeled Tomatoes
- 2 tablespoons balsamic vinegar
- 2 tablespoons cane sugar
- 1 tablespoon fresh thyme leaves
- 1/ 2 teaspoon salt
- 4 large eggs
- Salt, as needed
- Black pepper, as needed
- 4 tablespoons butter
- 4 slices sourdough, or country style bread
- 1/ 2 cup shredded mozzarella

Instructions

1. Over medium heat, add 14.5 oz can Muir Glen Organic Whole Peeled Tomatoes to a small sauce pan. Allow tomatoes to come to a simmer. Then, using a potato masher or a fork, carefully mash tomatoes in their juices. Let simmer another 5 minutes. Then, add balsamic vinegar, sugar, thyme and 1/2 teaspoon salt. Mix, and let mixture simmer about 25 minutes, stirring occasionally, until it has thickened. Remove jam from heat, and set it aside.

2. Using 3 tablespoons butter, spread butter over the outside of each slice of bread. Flip slices over, and add cheese to the inside of 2 of the slices.

3. Scramble eggs in a bowl with a pinch of salt and pepper. Heat the remaining butter over medium-low heat in a pan. After a minute or two, add the eggs, and allow them to cook, undisturbed, until a thin rim of cooked egg beginning to appear along the edges. Then, using a rubber spatula, continuously push the eggs in the pan until they are velvety and fluffy in texture and just set. Remove them from heat immediately, and set aside.

4. Layer eggs over the two slices of bread with the cheese. Then, scoop desired amount of tomato jam

onto the eggs. Add the top layer of bread, making sure the butter is on the outside.

5. Heat a skillet over medium heat, and cook each sandwich for about 4-5 minutes, flipping half way, so that both sandwiches are golden brown on each side. Remove from heat, carefully slice in half, and sprinkle with more fresh thyme leaves and sea salt. Serve and enjoy!

Prep Time: 10 Minutes

Cook Time: 15 Minutes

Servings: 4

Ingredients

- 1 sweet potato, washed, peeled and cubed
- Extra-virgin olive oil
- Salt, to taste
- Smoked paprika, to taste
- Chili lime seasoning, to taste
- 1/ 2 cup kaniwa
- 1 medium egg
- 2 large handfuls mixed greens
- Lemon juice
- Black pepper, to taste
- 1/ 2 avocado, sliced `
- Red pepper flakes, for garnish
- Hemp seeds, for garnish

Instructions

1. Preheat the oven to 400°F. Line a baking sheet with parchment paper.

2. Toss sweet potato with a drizzle of oil, salt, smoked paprika and chili lime seasoning. Spread in a single layer on the prepared baking sheet and roast for 30 minutes.

3. In a medium saucepan combine the kaniwa and 1 cup water. Bring to a boil, stir, and cover. Let simmer for about 15 minutes, until all the water has evaporated.

4. Meanwhile, bring a small pot filled with water to a rapid boil. Carefully lower the egg into the water and cook for 7 minutes. Immediately transfer egg to a bowl of ice and let cool completely. Peel and slice in half once cooled.

5. To assemble, layer the greens in a large bowl. Dress with a drizzle of oil, lemon juice, salt and pepper to taste. Add the cooked kaniwa, roasted sweet potatoes and egg. Garnish with red pepper flakes and hemp seeds.

Prep Time: 15 Minutes

Cook Time: 1hrs 35 Minutes

Servings: 1

Ingredients

For The Baked Beans:

- 2 15 ounce cans baked beans
- 1/ 4 cup packed brown sugar
- 1 onion, chopped
- 1/ 4 cup ketchup
- 1 tablespoon Dijon mustard
- 1 tablespoon Worcestershire sauce
- 1 teaspoon red wine vinegar
- Salt and pepper, to taste
- 3 slices crispy bacon, chopped
- For The Potatoes
- 1 potato, of your choice
- 1 tablespoon olive oil
- Salt and pepper, to taste

For The Tomatoes

- 1 beefsteak tomato

- 2 teaspoons olive oil

- Salt and pepper, to taste

For The Plate:

- 2 slices bacon

- 1 sausage

- 1/ 2 cup mushrooms, sliced

- 2 eggs

- 3 tablespoons butter, divided

- 1 slice brown bread or soda bread

Instructions

1. Make the baked beans: Preheat the oven to 350°F. Combine all ingredients in a 9-inch baking dish. Bake for 1 hour.

2. Make the tomatoes: Raise the oven to 425°F. Slice the tomato into 1/4-inch thick slices. Drizzle with olive oil and season with salt and pepper. Place on a parchment-lined baking sheet. Roast until softened and browned in spots, about 25 minutes.

3. Make the potatoes: Cut the potato into medium cubes. Drizzle with olive oil, season with salt and pepper,

then spread in an even layer on a parchment-lined baking sheet. Roast for 20 minutes, flipping halfway through.

4. Heat 1 tablespoon of butter int a cast-iron skillet on medium heat. Fry the bacon and sausage until crispy, about 3 minutes each side. Transfer to a plate. Add the mushrooms to the skillet and cook until soft, about 4 minutes. Transfer to the plate, then fry the eggs in the skillet, cooking for about 3-4 minutes until the whites are set and the yolks still runny. Add more butter to the skillet as needed.

5. Once everything is cooked, arrange it all on the plate with the bacon and mushrooms. Serve with a slice of bread.

Prep Time: 15 Minutes

Cook Time: 5 Minutes

Servings: 1

Ingredients

- 2 teaspoons instant coffee
- 1 tablespoon cocoa powder
- 2 teaspoons honey or maple syrup
- 1 1/ 2 cups granola
- 1/ 2 cup blueberries
- 1/ 2 cup raspberries
- 1 cup strawberries, halved
- 1 ounce vegan dark chocolate semisweet morsels
- 1 pieces medium banana, sliced
- 1 1/ 4 cup almond milk and coconut milk blend or other non-dairy milk alternative
- 2 tablespoons peanuts

Instructions

1. Bring 1 cup of water to a boil. Add cocoa powder and instant coffee to a medium bowl. Add hot water and stir a little until just combined, and then add the honey.
2. Whip the mixture with an electric beater or immersion blender with the whisk attachment, using a back and forth motion. This might take at least a few minutes to get a good pudding-like whipped consistency.
3. Pour some granola into a bowl, top with sliced banana, blueberries, raspberries, strawberries, peanuts and dark chocolate morsels. These ingredients are flexible, so use what you have at hand.
4. Scoop half of the whipped coffee chocolate "pudding" into the bowl.
5. Pour almond, coconut, soy, oat, or other non-dairy alternative into the bowl. Mix the whipped coffee cocoa into the other ingredients as it's strong on it's own!
6. Enjoy that energy and buzz!

11. Peanut Satay Noodles

Prep Time: 15 Minutes

Cook Time: 15 Minutes

Servings: 6

Ingredients

- 1 lb butternut squash , or kabocha squash
- 1 cup edamame
- 1 zucchini
- 1 bok choy , chopped (or handful spinach)
- 1 package brown rice noodles (250g)
- 1/4 cup peanuts , chopped (optional for topping)
- 4 green onion (optional for topping)
- 1-2 sprigs fresh basil (optional for topping)

Peanut Sauce Dressing:

- 1/3 cup all-natural peanut butter
- 1/3 cup coconut milk
- 1 tbsp sesame oil
- 2 tbsp tamari

- 1 tsp white miso
- 1 /2 tsp cayenne pepper flakes
- 1 lime juiced

Instructions

1. Make your peanut sauce: Add peanut butter, coconut milk, sesame oil, tamari, miso paste, cayenne flakes, and lime juice to a bowl. Whisk with fork to combine until smooth.

2. Preheat oven to 200C/400F. Cut squash into small bite sized pieces discarding the tough skin. (If using a kabocha squash you do not have to peel the skins, as they are soft and edible). Arrange onto a parchment lined baking tray and bake for 15 minutes, or until softened. Soak rice noodles in warm water for 10 minutes.* In a saucepan bring water to boil, add rice noodle and cook for approx. 5 minutes, or until al-dente. Strain, and reserve noodle water.

3. Spiralize zucchini into noodle shape. (Or grate, or chop into thin bite sized pieces). Toss zucchini into a saucepan and sauté on medium heat for 5 minutes, or until warm and just cooked. (Optional to add splashes

water, or 2 tsp neutral oil if needed to stop veg from sticking).

4. Add edamame and bok choy to saucepan. Stir until bok choy is wilted, approx. 1-2 minutes. Add the cooked squash, noodles and peanut sauce. Mix to combine. (Optional to add splashes of reserved noodle water to thin if sauce is too thick). Serve in bowls topped with chopped peanuts, green onion and fresh basil.

Prep Time: 1hrs 5 Minutes

Cook Time: 15 Minutes

Servings: 6

Ingredients

- 1 1/2 cup sushi rice
- 3 cup water
- 1 cup purple cabbage shredded
- 1 carrot
- 1 cup kale chopped
- 1 avocado
- 1/4 cup alfalfa sprouts
- 7 nori sheets
- Tamari Almond Butter Sauce:
- 1/4 cup almond butter
- 2 tbsp tamari
- 1/2 tsp white miso
- 1 lemon , juiced
- 1/4 tsp cayenne pepper flakes

- 3 tbsp water

Instructions

1. Begin by making sushi rice. Rinse rice thoroughly, then add to saucepan with water. Cook rice for 15 minutes, or as instructed on package. Remove from heat and fluff with a wooden spoon. Cover with tea towel and let cool long enough to be able to handle with your hands.

2. While you are waiting for the rice, prepare your veg. Thinly slice cabbage, and cut carrot into matchsticks (I recommend using a mandolin for this). Chop kale leaves into small pieces, discarding the stems. Thinly slice avocado.

3. Place bamboo sushi mat on work station (you can also use plastic wrap, if you don't have a bamboo sushi mat). Lay nori sheet on top of matt and gently press sushi rice on top to cover nori sheet in a thin layer.

4. Arrange veggies in an even layer (avocado, red cabbage, carrot, kale and alfalfa), parallel to the edge of the nori sheet, leaving about 1-inch of rice at the top undecorated. (for a visual, see image in blog post above)

5. Gently roll bamboo matt away from you, to roll the nori sheet into a log like a burrito. (For a tightly packed roll tuck in the veg with your fingers as you). Once in a roll, use a little bit of water to seal the edge.

6. Slice sushi roll into bite sized sushi pieces with a sharp knife and set aside. Continue this process until you've used all the rice, nori sheets and veg. (I was able to make 7 rolls).

7. To make the tamari almond butter sauce, add almond butter, tamari, miso, lemon juice, cayenne pepper flakes and water to a bowl. Whisk until smooth and creamy. Optional to add more water to thin if desired.

8. Tamari Almond Butter Sauce can be made ahead, it will last in fridge for up to 5 days.

9. Sushi will last in fridge for up to 24 hours. I recommend leaving in log form and covered well with wrap. Keep in the fridge. Cut into bite-sized sushi pieces before serving.

10. If you don't have a bamboo sushi mat you can use a square of plastic wrap. (I have never tried this but I imagine it's a bit more finicky).

Prep Time: 15 Minutes

Cook Time: 35 Minutes

Servings: 6

Ingredients

- 1 white onion diced
- 3 cloves garlic finely chopped
- 1 tsp coconut oil
- pinch sea salt
- 4 white potatoes medium, cubed
- 1/2 cauliflower chopped
- 10-12 cherry tomatoes
- 3 cups vegetable stock or water
- 2 tbsp tomato paste
- 1 1/2 tsp turmeric
- 1 1/2 tsp cumin
- 1 inch fresh ginger peeled and grated
- 1/2 lemon juiced
- 1/4 tsp cayenne pepper or to taste
- 1/2 cup dried red lentils
- 1 can coconut milk

- Sea salt and pepper to taste
- Fresh cilantro for topping

Instructions

1. In a large pot add chopped onion and garlic. Add 1 tsp coconut oil and a pinch sea salt and bring to medium-high heat. Cook onion and garlic stirring occasionally until onion turns translucent, approx. 10 minutes.

2. Add chopped potatoes to the pot and cook until they start to sweat, approx. 10 minutes. Then add cauliflower florets and cherry tomatoes. Pour in vegetable stock. Cover pot and bring to a simmer. Then add tomato paste, turmeric, cumin, freshly grated ginger, and lemon juice.

3. Pour in red lentils and simmer curry on medium-low heat for 15-20 minutes, or until lentils and veg are cooked and curry has thickened. Lastly, pour in coconut milk and stir to combine.

4. Add cayenne pepper, sea salt and pepper to taste. Serve curry with brown rice or naan bread.

Prep Time: 20 Minutes

Cook Time: 23 Minutes

Servings: 6

Ingredients

For The Kale Caesar Dressing:

- 1 1/2 lemons juiced
- 1/4 cup tahini
- 2 cloves garlic finely chopped
- pinch sea salt
- filtered water to thin (I used 2-3 tbsp)

Other Ingredients:

- 1 bunch kale (200 g/7 oz)
- 1/2 cup raw cashews
- 2 tbsp hemp hearts
- 1 apple thinly sliced
- 1/3 cup pomegranate seeds
- 2 tbsp dried cranberries
- 3 dates pits removed and chopped
- sea salt and pepper to taste

Instructions

1. Make your Kale Caesar Dressing: In a small bowl add lemon juice, tahini, chopped garlic, and sea salt. Whisk to combine. Add splashes of water to thin until desired dressing consistency (I used 2-3 tbsp).

2. Wash kale well. Tear leaves into small bite sized pieces and place in a large mixing bowl. Discard the stems. Pour dressing over kale leaves and toss to combine.

3. Roast cashews in saucepan on medium heat, stirring occasionally until cashews are browned, (approx. 6-8 minutes). Let cashews cool slightly then chop and sprinkle over kale salad. Add hemp hearts and toss to combine.

4. Transfer kale caesar salad into a serving bowl and top with sliced apple, pomegranate seeds, cranberries and chopped dates. Season with salt and pepper and serve

Prep Time: 20 Minutes

Cook Time: 35 Minutes

Servings: 4

Ingredients

- 1/2 cups brown rice uncooked
- 3 cups water
- 1 lb watermelon
- 2 peaches
- 1 heirloom tomato yellow or red
- 1 avocado
- 2 green onion finely chopped
- 1/4 cup fresh mint finely chopped
- Citrus Tamari Dressing:
- 2 lemons juiced
- 1/2 tsp ginger fresh and grated
- 1 1/2 tsp tamari
- 1 1/2 tsp maple syrup
- 1 tbsp sesame oil or olive oil

Instructions

1. In a pot add brown rice and water. Bring to a boil, then reduce heat to simmer and cook rice for 30 minutes, or as instructed on package. Remove from heat and fluff with a wooden spoon. Then, cover the pot with dish towel and secure with lid until ready to serve. (The dish towel will help to keep the rice fluffy).

2. Using a melon baller, scoop watermelon into round balls. (Or, cut into bite-sized cubes). Add to a large mixing bowl. Chop peaches, tomato and avocado into bite-sized pieces and add to bowl. Finely chop onion and fresh mint and add to bowl. Gently mix ingredients with hands to combine.

3. In a bowl add the juice of two lemons, freshly grated ginger, tamari, maple syrup and sesame oil. Whisk to combine. Drizzle watermelon poke mix with enough dressing to lightly coat, reserving the rest for serving. Scoop rice into bowls and top with watermelon poke. Drizzle with remaining Citrus Tamari Dressing.

Prep Time: 20 Minutes

Cook Time: 40 Minutes

Servings: 4

Ingredients

- 4 garlic cloves
- 2 onions
- 2 tbsp coconut oil
- 4.5cups carrots peeled and chopped
- 1 sweet potato peeled and chopped
- pinch sea salt
- 3 cups water
- 1 tsp fresh ginger grated
- 2 tbsp curry powder
- 1 tbsp coriander ground
- 1/2 tsp cayenne pepper flakes
- 1 can coconut milk (400 ml)
- 1/2 lemon juiced

Instructions

1. Dice onions and garlic, and add to a large pot with coconut oil. Bring pot to medium-low heat, and cook veg stirring occasionally for approx. 10 minutes, or until onion turns translucent.

2. Peel and cut carrots and sweet potato into roughly chopped chunks, and add to the pot. Add a pinch of salt. Cover pot with lid and let the vegetables sweat, stirring occasionally for 15 minutes, or until slightly softened.

3. Add water to the pot and bring soup to a simmer. Add grated ginger, curry powder, coriander, and cayenne pepper flakes. Season with sea salt and pepper and simmer soup on low heat for 20 minutes, or until veg is very soft.

4. Puree soup using a hand mixer, or a blender on low, until completely smooth.

5. Stir in coconut cream, and add more spices, salt and pepper if desired. Optional to add splashes more water to thin if desired.

6. Transfer soup to bowls and serve.

Prep Time: 30 Minutes

Cook Time: 40 Minutes

Servings: 6

Ingredients

For The Crust:

- 1/4 cup chia seeds ground
- 1/2 cup water
- 2 cups cauliflower shredded
- 1/2 cup almond meal
- 1/2 cup buckwheat flour
- 2 tbsp nutritional yeast
- 2 cloves garlic finely chopped
- 1 tsp onion powder
- 1 tsp sea salt
- 1 tsp pepper

For The Cashew Parsley Pesto:

- 2 cups parsley
- 1 cup cashews
- 1/2 cup olive oil

- 1 lemon juiced
- Additional Toppings:
- 1 cup cherry tomatoes
- 1 tbsp olive oil plus more if needed
- 1/2 cup kale chopped
- 1/4 cup radish thinly sliced
- 1/4 cup pomegranate seeds

Instructions

1. Preheat oven to 400F/200C. Make chia egg by adding whisking together ground chia and water. Let absorb for at least 10 minutes.

2. In a food processor pulse cauliflower until it shredded. (Or grate by hand). Then add to a large mixing bowl with almond meal, buckwheat flour, chia egg, nutritional yeast, garlic, onion powder, salt and pepper. Knead with your hands to create a large doughy ball.

3. Line a baking tray with parchment paper and transfer dough on top. Roll it out to be 1/4 inch thick. Bake for 30 minutes or until golden. Remove from oven and place on a cooling rack.

4. Meanwhile, make your cashew parsley pesto: In a food processor add parsley, cashews, oil and lemon. Pulse until combined.

5. Paint cherry tomatoes with oil and cook in oven on broil for 10 minutes, or until bursted and slightly charred.

6. Lather flatbread with pesto and top with roasted tomatoes, chopped kale, radish, and pomegranate.

Prep Time: 20 Minutes

Cook Time: 10 Minutes

Servings: 6

Ingredients

- 1 cup quinoa uncooked (I used tricolour quinoa)
- 2 cup water
- 1 red onion small
- 2 celery stalks
- 1 1/2 cup cherry tomatoes (300g/10 oz)
- 1/2 cup parsley tightly packed
- 1/2 cup dill tightly packed
- 1 can chickpeas (400 ml/14 fl oz)
- 1/4 cup pumpkin seeds

Lemon Vinaigrette Dressing:

- 1/4 cup olive oil + 1 tbsp
- 3 tbsp lemon juice
- 1 clove garlic finely chopped
- Sea salt pinch
- Pepper pinch

Instructions

1. In a saucepan combine quinoa and water. Bring to a boil, then reduce to simmer and cook quinoa for 12-15 minutes. Fluff with a spoon and cover with tea towel. Let rest.
2. Dice onion, and chop celery and tomatoes into small chunks. Finely chop parsley and dill. Drain and rinse chickpeas.
3. In a large mixing bowl combine quinoa with veg, herbs, chickpeas and pumpkin seeds.
4. Prepare vinaigrette: in a small mixing bowl combine olive oil, lemon juice, chopped garlic, sea salt and pepper. Whisk to combine. Pour lemon vinaigrette over quinoa salad and toss to combine.

Prep Time: 50 Minutes

Cook Time: 50 Minutes

Servings: 4

Ingredients

- Homemade Enchilada Sauce (Makes 1.5 Cups):
- 3 tbsp neutral oil (avocado oil or coconut oil)
- 3 tbsp all-purpose flour , or gluten-free
- 1.5tsp chili powder
- 1/2 tsp garlic powder
- 1 tsp cumin
- 1/4 tsp cayenne pepper flakes
- 1/8 tsp cinnamon
- 1/2 tsp sea salt
- 1/8 tsp ground black pepper
- 2 tbsp tomato paste
- 1.5 cups vegetable broth
- 1 tsp apple cider vinegar

Enchilada Stuffing:

- 2 sweet potatoes

- 2 tbsp neutral oil (avocado oil or coconut oil)
- 1 onion (red or white), chopped
- 3 cloves garlic , finely chopped
- 1 red bell pepper , chopped
- 1 tbsp neutral oil (avocado oil or coconut oil)
- 1 tsp cumin
- 1/2 tsp sea salt
- 1/2 tsp chili powder
- 1/4 tsp cinnamon
- 2 cups baby spinach , tightly packed
- 1 can black beans (14 fl oz/400 ml), strained and rinsed
- 6 8-inch whole-wheat flour tortillas (or gluten-free tortillas)
- Cilantro Lime Avocado Crema:
- 3/4 cup coconut yogurt
- 1 avocado
- 1/2 cup cilantro , tightly packed
- 1/4 cup lime juice
- 1 clove garlic
- 1/4 tsp sea salt

Instructions

2. Homemade Enchilada Sauce (Makes 1.5 Cups)

3. Measure out all your dry ingredients, as well as tomato paste and veg broth. The recipe comes together quickly, so have them close by.

4. Heat oil in a medium-sized saucepan on high. Once hot (i.e. the surface is shimmering) whisk in all-purpose flour and spice mixture. Continue whisking to combine, until thick and fragrant. Then add tomato paste.

5. Slowly splash in vegetable broth. Continue whisking to form a smooth liquid. Bring sauce to a low simmer and cook for 5 to 10 mins, or until thick and saucy. (Consistency should be thick like ketchup). Splash in apple cider vinegar and stir to combine. Remove from heat and cover.

Enchiladas

1. Preheat oven to 400F/200C. Chop sweet potatoes into bite-sized cubes. Line a baking tray with parchment paper and spread sweet potatoes onto tray. Drizzle with oil and toss to coat. Cook for 20 mins. (Keep oven on for later).

2. Meanwhile, toss onion, garlic, red bell pepper, and 1 tbsp neutral oil into a large deep skillet (or saucepan) on medium-high heat. Cook, stirring often until veg is softened (approx. 10 mins). Then add cumin, sea salt, chili powder and cinnamon. Toss to combine.

3. Drop in spinach and cook for a few minutes until wilted. Finish by dropping in roasted sweet potato and black beans. Stir to combine. Remove from heat.

4. Assemble enchiladas by pouring 1/4 cup of the homemade enchilada sauce into your casserole dish. (I used a 8.5 x 11 inch baking dish). Spread out the sauce to coat the base.

5. Grab a tortilla and add spoonfuls of filling mixture to the middle. You want it full, but not too full that you can't roll it (about 1/2 cup of filling should do). Snugly fold in the sides to form a log. Place the burrito seam side down into your casserole dish. Repeat with remaining tortillas and filling, until you've used them all up and the tortillas are snug in the casserole dish,

6. Drizzle the top of your pan with remaining homemade enchilada sauce. Spread to cover as best you can. Cook enchiladas for 20 mins, or until the top is golden and bubbling. Let cool slightly (approx. 10 mins) before serving.

Cilantro Lime Avocado Crema:

1. Meanwhile, prepare your crema by adding all the contents to a blender. Blend until smooth and creamy. Drizzle enchilada casserole with the avocado crema. Optional to sprinkle casserole with more cilantro. Serve enchiladas with remaining crema.

Prep Time: 5hrs 50 Minutes

Cook Time: 20 Minutes

Servings: 4

Ingredients

- 3 3/4 cups all purpose flour plus 1/2 to 1 cup more
- 1 1/2 cups filtered water
- 2 teaspoons sea salt finely ground
- 1/4 teaspoon active dry yeast
- Sauce and Toppings:
- 1 cup tomato sauce
- 1 tbsp tomato paste
- 2 cloves garlic finely chopped
- pinch sea salt
- 1 cup Homemade Vegan Mozzarella or store-bought
- 1/2 cup basil fresh, finely chopped

Instructions

2. In a large mixing bowl, combine flour, salt, and yeast. Gradually add 1.5 cups water while stirring with a

wooden spoon. Stir until well incorporated. Knead dough gently with your hands to form a dough ball. Add more flour if needed until it's no longer sticky to the touch. It should be plush and dough-like. (I used about 1/2 cup more flour).

3. Transfer dough to a large clean bowl. Cover with reusable wrap and let dough rise at room temperature, in a draft-free area, until its surface is covered with tiny bubbles and the dough has doubled in size, approx. 6-10 hours. (I like to do this overnight).

4. If not using right away, dust dough ball with flour and cover in reusable wrap. Store in fridge and bring back to room temperature before use.

5. Transfer dough to a floured work surface and gently shape into a rough rectangle. Divide into two equal portions and mold each gently into a ball.

6. Preheat oven to 450F/230C. Place dough balls each on a rimmed baking sheet and flatten with hands, until it covers most of the sheet. (If the dough springs back, let it rest a few minutes, then try again).

Sauce and Toppings:

1. In a smaller mixing bowl combine tomato sauce, tomato paste, garlic and sea salt. Slather tomato sauce onto pizza dough and top each with vegan mozzarella.

2. Bake pizzas for 15 to 20 minutes, or until pizza crust is golden and bubbly, and the bottom is cooked through (golden and crispy - check by lifting up the pizza with a spatula and peeking underneath). Sprinkle pizza with fresh basil and slice into 8 pieces.

21. Easy Zucchini Lasagna

Prep Time: 30 Minutes

Cook Time: 1hrs 20 Minutes

Servings: 8

Ingredients

- 3 zucchini
- 3 cups vegan mozzarella , grated (optional)

Vegan Bolognese:

- 4 cloves garlic
- 2.75 cups tomato sauce
- 2 tbsp tomato paste
- 1 lemon , juiced (about 4 tbsp)
- pinch sea salt
- 1.5 cups green lentils , cooked
- Vegan Cheese Sauce:
- 1 cup raw cashews , soaked overnight and strained
- 1/4 cup nutritional yeast
- 4 cloves garlic

- 1 lemon , juiced (approx. 4 tbsp)
- 1 cup water , plus more if needed
- 1 tsp onion powder (optional)
- 1/4 tsp salt

Instructions

2. Using a mandolin thinly slice zucchinis to be 1/8 inch thick. Lay out onto paper towel sheets. Place more paper towel on top and gently press the water out of zucchini as best you can.

3. Turn oven to broil and line baking tray with parchment paper. Lay zucchini slices onto tray without crowding, and place in oven for 3 minutes. (You might have to do this in a few batches so as not to overcrowd the tray). Remove and gently flip zucchini slices to bake other side, place back in the oven for another 2 minutes. (This will help to get more moisture out of the zucchini as they contain a lot of water). Remove from oven and let cool slightly, then gently pat out any excess moisture with paper towel.

4. To make your vegan Bolognese: Finely chop garlic and add to a saucepan with tomato sauce, tomato paste,

lemon juice and a generous pinch of salt. Bring to a simmer. Pulse lentils in blender (or food processor) and add to a saucepan. Cook sauce for 30 minutes until thick, and liquid is reduced by almost half.

5. Make your homemade vegan sauce. In a blender add soaked cashews (strained), nutritional yeast, garlic, lemon juice, water, onion powder (optional) and salt. Blend until creamy and smooth.

6. Turn oven to 375F/190C, and build your lasagna: In a 8×11 casserole, spread a thin even layer of vegan Bolognese on the bottom and layer the zucchini on top to cover. Pour a thin layer of homemade vegan cheese sauce over top of zucchini. Then sprinkle with a thin layer of vegan mozzarella cheese. Repeat the process until all your ingredients are used up (ending with the vegan mozzarella cheese, or homemade vegan cheese sauce).

7. Cover with foil and bake zucchini lasagna for 30 minutes. Then remove foil and bake for another 20 minutes. Let lasagna sit for 10-15 minutes before serving.

Prep Time: 30 Minutes

Cook Time: 20 Minutes

Servings: 6

Ingredients

- 0.5-1 cup gluten-free oats
- 3 cloves garlic , diced
- 1 small white onion , diced
- 1 tbsp coconut oil
- 5 cups cremini mushrooms , sliced (1 large box)
- 1 cup chickpeas
- 2 tsp gluten-free tamari
- 1/2 lemon , juiced
- 2 tbsp almond butter
- 3 tbsp nutritional yeast
- 1 tsp cumin
- 1 tsp paprika
- 1/4 tsp sea salt
- pinch pepper
- 1/2 cup parsley , chopped and tightly packed
- vegan gravy , to drizzle

Instructions

1. In your food processor add oats, pulse into a flour-like substance. Remove from food processor and place to the side.

2. In a skillet add diced garlic and onion with coconut oil. Bring to medium heat and add mushrooms. Cook stirring often until browned and ready to eat (10-15 minutes). Transfer to food processor along with 1/2 cup oats, chickpeas, tamari, lemon juice, almond butter, nutritional yeast, cumin, paprika, sea salt and pepper. Blend until smooth and combined.

3. Next add remaining 1/2 cup oats in batches. Blend and check consistency, if too sticky add more oats to the mixture. You should be able to form into rough balls with a spoon (I used 1 cup ground oats in total.). Finally, add in chopped parsley and pulse until combined. Cover falafel mix and chill in fridge for at least one hour. (This will make forming balls easier).

4. Preheat oven to 375F/190C..Line a baking tray with parchment paper and scoop rounded tablespoon amounts of dough onto parchment paper, and gently form balls. (I used a spoon to do this). Bake falafels for 20-25 minutes, or until golden brown. Optional to drizzle with my Quick and Easy Vegan Gravy

Prep Time: 15 Minutes

Cook Time: 40 Minutes

Servings: 6

Ingredients

- 4 sweet potatoes
- 1 tbsp neutral oil (optional)
- 2 avocados
- 1/2 lemon , juiced
- pinch sea salt
- 2 green onions
- 2 cups white beans

Signature Citrus Tahini Dressing:

- 2 tbsp tahini
- 1/2 lemon , juiced
- pinch sea salt
- water , to thin (I used about 2 tbsp)

Instructions

1. Turn oven to 400F/200C. Using a fork, poke small holes in sweet potatoes going all the way round, about 1-inch apart. Line baking tray with parchment paper, and place sweet potatoes on top. Bake for 40 minutes, or until cooked through.
2. Mash avocado in a bowl with lemon juice and a pinch of sea salt. Finely chop green onion.
3. To make the citrus tahini dressing: combine tahini, lemon juice and a pinch sea salt in a bowl. Mix together to combine, then add splashes of water until you've reached desired consistency, (I used about 2 tbsp).
4. Cut sweet potatoes in half and fill with white beans, and mashed avocado. Sprinkle with green onion, and drizzle with citrus tahini dressing.
5. Sweet Potato

Prep Time: 10 Minutes

Cook Time: 20 Minutes

Servings: 4

Ingredients

Alfredo Sauce:

- 1 cup raw cashews , soaked overnight
- 1/4 cup nutritional yeast
- 3 cloves garlic
- 1.5 lemons , juiced (approx. 4 tbsp)
- 1 cup water , plus more if needed
- 1 tsp onion powder (optional)
- 1/4 tsp salt

For The Noodle Dish:

- 3 sweet potatoes , peeled and spiralized (about 1kg)
- 4 tsp coconut oil
- 300 g asparagus (1 bunch)
- 1 cup baby spinach
- 10 sun-dried tomatoes , chopped

Instructions

1. Begin by making your vegan alfredo sauce. In a blender add soaked cashews* (strained), nutritional yeast, garlic, lemon juice, water, onion powder (optional) and salt. Blend until creamy and smooth.

2. If you haven't already, peel and spiralize your sweet potatoes into thin noodles. Chop the white ends off asparagus and discard, keeping the fresh green tips. Then chop green tips into bite sized chunks.

3. In a skillet add 2 tsp (10 ml) coconut oil, bring to medium high heat. Add baby spinach and chopped asparagus, cook until spinach has wilted and asparagus has gone bright green in colour (3-5 minutes). Pour into a bowl and set aside.

4. Add 2 tsp more coconut oil to skillet and add spiralized sweet potato noodles. Cook sweet potato on medium high heat, until sweet potato noodles begins to soften and are almost al-dente (8-10 minutes).

5. Pour vegan alfredo sauce into pan and toss to combine. Continue cooking sweet potatoes until sauce has thickened and sweet potatoes are al-dente (approx. 5 more minutes). Optional to add splashes more water to thin the sauce if desired. Add the sautéed spinach and asparagus to the dish as well as

chopped sun-dried tomatoes, mix to combine. Scoop sweet potato alfredo noodles into bowls and serve.

Prep Time: 1hrs 10 Minutes

Cook Time: 20 Minutes

Servings: 12

Ingredients

- 1 1/2 cup sushi rice
- 3 cup water
- 1 cup purple cabbage , shredded
- 1 carrot
- 1/2 cucumber
- 1 avocado

For The Almond Butter Tamari Sauce:

- 1/4 cup almond butter
- 2 tbsp tamari
- 1/2 tsp miso white shiro
- 1 lemon , juiced
- 1/4 tsp cayenne pepper
- 3 tbsp filtered water

Instructions

1. Begin by making sushi rice. Rinse rice thoroughly, then add to saucepan with water. Cook rice for 15 minutes, or as instructed on package. Remove from heat and fluff with a wooden spoon. Cover with tea towel and let cool long enough to be able to handle with your hands.

2. While you are waiting for the rice, prepare your veg. Thinly slice cabbage and cucumber, and cut carrot into matchsticks (I recommend using a mandolin for this). Thinly slice avocado with a sharp knife.

3. Using a donut mould, mould the rice into donut shape. If you don't have a donut mould pack the sushi into a ball with your hands. Slightly flatten onto your work station, and stick your thumb into the centre of the ball to make an 'O' shape. (Lightly wet hands with water to stop the sushi from sticking to your hands. I did this throughout).

4. Decorate each donut with thin slices of cabbage, cucumber, carrots, and avocado to cover. Serve with tamari, or tamari almond butter sauce to dip.

5. To make the tamari almond butter sauce, add almond butter, tamari, miso, lemon juice, cayenne pepper

flakes and water to a bowl. Whisk until smooth and creamy. Optional to add more water to thin if desired.

Prep Time: 20 Minutes

Cook Time: 20 Minutes

Servings: 5

Ingredients

- 1/4 cup old-fashioned rolled oats
- 1/2 cup fresh parsley
- 6 cloves garlic
- 1 small onion
- 1 can chickpeas (strained and rinsed)
- 2 tbsp nutritional yeast
- 2 tbsp tahini
- 1/2 lemon juiced
- 1 tbsp olive oil
- 1/2 tsp ground cumin
- 1/2 tsp ground coriander
- 1/4 tsp ground cardamom
- 1/2 tsp sea salt
- 1/4 tsp pepper
- pinch cayenne pepper
- 2 tbsp olive oil (for painting)

For The Citrus Tahini Dressing:

- 1/4 cup tahini
- 2 lemons juices
- pinch salt
- filtered water , to thin (I used 2-3 tbsp)
- 5 whole-grain tortilla wraps
- 1 cup mixed greens of choice
- 1 cup purple cabbage , thinly sliced
- 1/2 cup cucumber , thinly sliced
- 2 avocados , thinly sliced

Instructions

1. In your food processor add oats, pulse into a flour-like substance. Remove from food processor and place to the side.
2. Next add parsley, garlic and onion to food processor. Pulse until finely chopped. Then add oat flour, chickpeas, nutritional yeast, tahini, lemon juice, olive oil, cumin, coriander, cardamom, sea salt, pepper and a pinch cayenne pepper. Pulse until it becomes a crumbly dough-like texture.

3. Transfer falafel dough to mixing bowl. Preheat oven to 375F/190C. Line a baking tray with parchment paper and scoop rounded tablespoon amounts of dough onto parchment paper, and gently form balls. (I used an ice cream scoop to do this.)

4. Paint falafels with a bit of olive oil and place in the oven to bake for 15-20 minutes, or until golden in colour.

5. To make the Citrus Tahini Sauce: in a bowl add tahini, lemon juice and salt. Mix to combine. Add splashes of water to thin until you've reached desired consistency. (I used 2-3 tbsp). Drizzle falafels with tahini sauce for eating.

6. To make the wraps combine mixed greens, cabbage, cucumber, avocado and 2-3 falafels in a whole wheat tortilla wrap, drizzle with citrus tahini dressing and serve.

Prep Time: 10 Minutes

Cook Time: 15 Minutes

Servings: 10

Ingredients

- 1/2 cup warm water
- 1 teaspoon coconut sugar
- 1 packet active dry yeast
- 2 3/4 cups all-purpose flour (+ 1/2-3/4 more for kneading)
- 1/3 cup vegan butter melted
- 1/2 cup unsweetened almond milk
- 1/3 cup coconut sugar
- 1 teaspoon fine sea salt
- 1 tbsp neutral oil
- 1/2 cup vegan butter
- 2/3 cup coconut sugar
- 2 tbsp cinnamon

Instructions

1. In a small bowl add warm water. Stir in coconut sugar until mostly dissolved. Then add yeast and stir. Set aside for about 7 minutes, or until yeast is dissolved and liquid mixture creates foamy bubbles on top.

2. (If bubbles do not form, toss and try again. Water should be warm but not boiling or it will kill the yeast).

3. Add 2 cups flour to a large mixing bowl. In a separate mixing bowl, combine melted butter, almond milk, coconut sugar, and sea salt. Pour in yeast mixture and stir to combine.

4. Pour wet mixture over your flour and stir with a large wooden spoon. Mix until combined and resembling batter consistency. Then add remaining 3/4 cups flour. Mix together.

5. Knead mixture until it comes together in a shaggy and sticky dough. Flour work surface and place dough on top. Knead the dough, adding small handfuls of flour as needed, until it's no longer sticky to the touch, approx. 3-4 minutes. The dough should be smooth and elastic. (Don't be afraid to add lots more flour. Adding 1/2 cup to 3/4 cups while kneading is normal).

When dough is no longer sticky to the touch, shape it into a big ball.

6. Wash mixing bowl and dry it. Lightly oil the bowl with 1 tbsp neutral oil (or melted vegan butter) and place dough inside. Flip the dough around so it gets lightly coated in the oil. Then, tightly cover the bowl with bees wrap and place in a draft-free area. Let the dough rise for at least 1 hour. (It should almost double in size).

7. Meanwhile, make the cinnamon sugar filling. In a small bowl combine vegan butter, coconut sugar and cinnamon. Set aside.

8. When dough has risen, divide it into 2 equal portions (to make 2 dough balls). Place on a clean work surface to the side.

9. Preheat oven to 400F (200C). On a floured work surface, taking one dough ball at at a time, roll the dough into a rectangle as best you can, about 1/8 inch thick. Don't worry if it's not a perfect rectangle, my edges were wiggly.

10. Lather cinnamon filling over dough in an even layer, leaving a clean 1/2-inch border around the edges. Then roll the dough away from you to form a log.

11. Rotate log so that the end side is nearest you and using a sharp knife, cut the log in half vertically (from top to bottom) leaving about 1/2 inch at the top uncut.

12. Start braiding the two pieces, one over the other, trying to keep the open layers exposed so the cut side remains on top (this is what makes this braid effect). When you've braided the entire log pinch the ends together, and form a circular wreath. Gently transfer braided cinnamon wreath to a baking sheet lined with parchment paper.

13. Rolling out your second dough ball, and continue steps for lathering with cinnamon filling, rolling, slicing and braiding. Forming a wreath. Place on same baking tray, ensuring there is at least 2-3 inches between both wreaths. They will expand as they cook. (If you have remaining cinnamon filling you can serve with cinnamon buns as a buttery spread)

14. Bake cinnamon buns for 15-20 minutes, or until golden brown. Serve warm with remaining cinnamon filling.

Prep Time: 1hrs Minutes

Cook Time: 15 Minutes

Servings: 3

Ingredients

- 3 3/4 cup all-purpose flour plus more for shaping dough
- 1 1/2 cup water
- 2 tsp sea salt finely ground
- 1/4 tsp active dry yeast

Toppings:

- 1 can tomato sauce (400ml/13.5 oz)
- 3 cloves garlic finely chopped
- 1 zucchini thinly sliced
- 1 cup mushrooms thinly sliced
- 1 cup grape tomatoes halved
- 1 red onion small. thinly sliced
- 1/2 cup chickpeas
- pinch sea salt
- pinch pepper

- 1/4 cup basil chopped, tightly packed

Instructions

1. Whisk flour, salt, and yeast in a large mixing bowl. Gradually add 1.5 cups water while stirring with a wooden spoon. Stir until well incorporated.
2. Knead dough with hands to bring it together and form into a rough ball. Add more flour if needed until it's no longer sticky to the touch, or alternatively more water if it's too dry. It should be plush and dough-like. (I added 1/2 cup more flour).
3. Transfer dough to a large clean bowl. Cover with bees wrap and let dough rise at room temperature, in a draft-free area, until its surface is covered with tiny bubbles and the dough has doubled in size, approx. 6-10 hours. (I like to leave mine overnight).
4. Transfer dough to a floured work surface and gently shape into a rough rectangle. Divide into three equal portions and mould portions gently into a ball. Dust dough balls with more flour, and cover with bees wrap until ready to use. Bring dough back to room temperate before baking.

To Make Pizza

1. Preheat oven to 240C/475F. Place dough ball on a rimmed baking sheet. Flatten dough with hands, until it covers most of the sheet. You want it to be thin. (If dough springs back, let it rest a few minutes, then try again).

2. Mix tomato sauce, garlic, salt and pepper in a bowl. Paint sauce over the pizza dough leaving approx. 1 inch for the crust.

3. Decorate pizza with sliced zucchini, mushrooms, cherry tomatoes, and red onion. Sprinkle with salt and pepper and cook for 10-12 mins, or until bottom is crisp and top is slightly blistered. Remove from oven and sprinkle with chickpeas, more sea salt and pepper, and fresh basil leaves. Cut into 8 slices and serve.

4. Continue steps for making pizza for remaining 2 pizza doughs.

Prep Time: 15Minutes

Cook Time: 30 Minutes

Servings: 4

Ingredients

Buddha Bowl:

- 1 cup brown rice
- 2 cups water
- 1 cup corn chopped
- 1 cup pineapple chopped
- 1 yellow pepper chopped
- 1/2 cup yellow cherry tomatoes halved
- 1/2 cup raw cashews chopped
- 3 tbsp hemp hearts

Dressing:

- 1/3 cup tahini
- 1/4 cup water as needed for thinning
- 1/4 cup lemon juice plus more if desired
- 1/4 tsp sea salt

Instructions

1. In a saucepan add your brown rice and water. Bring to a boil, then reduce to simmer and cook for 30 minutes, or as instructed on package.

2. In a bowl add cooked rice, corn, pineapple, yellow peppers, cherry tomatoes, cashews and hemp hearts.

3. Prepare your dressing by whisking together tahini, water, lemon juice and sea salt in a bowl. Drizzle over buddha bowl and toss to combine.

Prep Time: 15 Minutes

Cook Time: 20 Minutes

Servings: 4

Ingredients

- 1 cup cherry tomatoes
- 1 tbsp avocado oil or other neutral oil
- 1 packet pasta of choice (500g)
- 1/3 cup olive oil
- 1/4 cup lemon juice
- 1 cup corn
- 1 cup chickpeas
- 1/4 cup chives chopped
- 1/4 cup fresh parsley chopped
- 1/4 cup mint leaves chopped
- 1/4 cup basil chopped
- 1/4 tsp sea salt
- 1/4 tsp cayenne pepper optional

Instructions

1. Preheat oven to 200C /400F. Paint cherry tomatoes with avocado oil and bake for 15 mins, or until bright and bursted. Remove from oven and place to the side.

2. Bring a large pot of water to a boil. Add noodles and cook spaghetti until just al-dente (approx. 5 minutes). Strain noodles.

3. Transfer noodles back to pot and drizzle with olive oil and lemon juice. Add tomatoes and corn, chickpeas, and chopped chives, parsley, mint and basil. Sprinkle with sea salt and cayenne (optional). Toss to combine.

www.ingramcontent.com/pod-product-compliance
Lightning Source LLC
Chambersburg PA
CBHW050838260726
48660CB00006B/2314